THE POWER AND POTENTIAL OF CHELATION

Chelation therapy is a noninvasive treatment for vascular disease that has been used since the 1950s with great success. It is the intravenous administration of a synthetic amino acid that binds with heavy metals and removes them from the system. By so doing, it reduces free radical damage to blood vessels and other tissues and helps improve circulation throughout the body. Besides benefit to people with vascular disease, chelation can reduce the risk of developing many chronic degenerative diseases, especially those related to free-radical damage such as cancer, inflammatory joint disease, asthma, diabetes, senile dementia and degenerative eye disease. Although the weight of clinical and scientific evidence, accumulating slowly over the past 45 years, clearly favors the use of chelation, the therapy remains controversial. Learn why, as Dr. Janson explains the basics of modern chelation therapy, the bias of the medical profession vs. the positive facts, treatment protocol, and the importance of using chelation as part of a comprehensive health program including nutrition and diet, dietary supplements, exercise and stress management.

ABOUT THE AUTHOR

Michael Janson, M.D. is president of the American College for Advancement in Medicine, and past-president of the American Preventive Medical Association. Dr. Janson lectures internationally on nutrition, alternative medicine, chelation therapy, and vitamins and other dietary supplements in medical therapy. He has testified twice before the U.S. Senate Labor and Human Resources Committee on the Dietary Supplement Act and the Access to Medical Treatment Act. In addition, he writes extensively for newsletters, journals and magazines such as *Alternative and Complementary Therapies, Nutrition Science News, New Age Journal* and the *Journal of Cardiovascular Nursing,* and is the author of the book, *The Vitamin Revolution in Health Care.* Dr. Janson maintains a private medical practice in Barnstable, Massachusetts, on Cape Cod.

Chelation Therapy and Your Health

This noninvasive treatment for vascular disease reduces free radical damage to blood vessels and helps improve circulation

Michael Janson, M.D.

K

KEATS PUBLISHING

LOS ANGELES

NTC/Contemporary Publishing Group

Chelation Therapy and Your Health is not intended as medical advice. Its intent is solely informational and educational. Please consult a health professional should the need for one be indicated.

CHELATION THERAPY AND YOUR HEALTH

ISBN 0-87983-899-X

Printed in United States of America

03 04 05 RCP 10 9 8 7 6 5 4

CONTENTS

INTRODUCTION

In the mid-1980s, I first saw Richard F., a mid-fifties business man who had recently told his golf partners that, because of his health, he would not make it to the next golf season. He had been suffering from chest pain and shortness of breath with the least activity, in spite of heart surgery a few years before. Now he could not even make it from the golf cart to the tee without problems. Prior to his visiting my office, Richard had accompanied a friend to visit a clinic in a neighboring state where the patients were receiving an intravenous therapy for their heart disease. After listening to their stories he told the doctor, "Hey, I gotta have some of that stuff." The doctor referred him to me because my office was much closer to his home.

It was clear from his medical history that Richard's chest pain, or angina pectoris, and shortness of breath were due to a recurrence of the hardening of the arteries (atherosclerosis or arteriosclerosis) to his heart. He did not want repeat bypass surgery, which had been recommended to him, but was taking some medications that had helped a little. He was overweight, paid little attention to diet, and his only physical activity was golf three or four times a month. He had smoked in the past but had given it up at the time of his earlier surgery. I suggested a course of treatment with intravenous chelation therapy, which was the treatment he had seen in the other office, and he agreed.

Richard also agreed to try to clean up his diet by reducing the fat and meat in it, reducing sugars, and eating more vegetables and fruits, whole grains and beans. I recommended dietary supplements as part of his health program, including vitamins E and C, magnesium and coenzyme Q10.

In a few weeks, Richard started to feel much better. He was able to walk farther without pain and he had much more energy. I cautioned him that for lasting benefits he had to change his diet and lose some weight, but he admitted that he found this difficult. His initial course of treatment lasted 18 weeks, and he had 36 chelation treatments in that time. His progress was remarkable although he lost little weight and still indulged in dietary excesses.

Richard's experience is similar to that of many other patients that I have treated with chelation therapy since 1983, and it is similar to what research and the clinical experience of many of my colleagues indicate. Although it has been around for nearly fifty years, chelation therapy is still a controversial treatment for blood vessel diseases. Just what is this treatment and how can it benefit people with vascular disease and a variety of other health problems? The importance of this question is underscored by the fact that heart and other blood vessel diseases are still the primary cause of death in the United States and other industrialized countries.

THE BASICS: WHAT IS CHELATION?

To start with the basics, a chelating agent is a substance that binds with metals and minerals because of its structure and bonding properties. Strictly speaking, chelation is defined as the incorporation of a metal ion into a heterocyclic ring structure. A chelating substance acts like a "claw," grabbing on to a metal atom, which is where is gets it name: *chele* is the Greek word for "claw." Chelating substances are well known in human and plant metabolism: heme, a part of hemoglobin, is a chelating substance that binds with iron, and magnesium is bound in chlorophyll as a chelate. The process of chelation is essential in human physiology for many enzyme reactions.

The absorption of nutrient minerals is dependent on chelation by transport proteins in the digestive tract.

Chelation therapy, as used for vascular disease, is a series of intravenous treatments with an amino acid called ethylene diamine tetraacetic acid, more commonly referred to as EDTA. Amino acids are the building block molecules of proteins, but EDTA is a synthetic amino acid that does not become incorporated into protein chains. In the 1930s, EDTA was developed as an industrial chelating agent to remove mineral deposits from machinery.

EDTA is used in foods as a preservative, and also in laboratory medicine. In foods, it binds with minerals to protect the food from spoilage and maintain the green color of frozen vegetables. In the lab, it is used as an anticlotting agent because it binds with calcium which is a necessary component in the clotting process. These uses require only very small amounts of EDTA to be effective. Eating the amount of EDTA used in foods probably has no physiological effect, partly because only a very small percentage of ingested EDTA will be absorbed, although it might decrease the absorption of some minerals from the intestinal tract.

Around 1950 EDTA was first administered to humans in an attempt to remove excessive lead. It worked and soon became the treatment of choice for lead toxicity. Heavier metals, such as lead, have a greater affinity for EDTA and form stronger bonds with it than do other, lighter-weight elements. EDTA also binds with nutritionally important elements such as calcium, iron, zinc, copper, manganese and others (the current protocol for treatment includes replacement of these elements with supplements).

Treatment with intravenous EDTA chelation helps many patients with a variety of diseases. Literature reports show possible benefits that go far beyond its role in heavy metal toxicity. For example, it helps to lower cholesterol levels, an effect reported as far back as 1955.[1] It has been reported to help with a metabolic disorder called porphyria,[2,3] in which abnormal metabolites are associated with digestive, skin, neurological and psychiatric symptoms. Chelation therapy can bring remarkable relief in patients with scleroderma,[4,5] a progressive hardening of the skin and other tissues, considered to be an autoimmune disease. Scleroderma is also known as systemic sclerosis. More recently, Dr. Elmer Cranton reports that he has seen remarkable improvement in his patients with scleroderma when treated with EDTA chelation. He says, "Nothing is better for scleroderma; nothing is even close to the benefits from EDTA. I have seen it do wonders with no failures."[6] How it helps these conditions is not known although there was quite a bit of speculation regarding mineral metabolism when these studies were first reported. Unfortunately, there has been little research into the value of chelation in these diseases since the 1950s.

In one series of thirty-two patients with rheumatoid arthritis, there was excellent improvement in 25 percent of the patients, and good improvement in 40 percent. Adding in the small group with fair improvement, the overall success rate was reported as 84 percent.[7] Many patients report that their arthritis symptoms improved after a series of chelation treatments. The few studies that have been done on arthritis and chelation confirm this clinical experience.

Although EDTA chelation therapy is accepted as a treatment for a number of health problems, it is most widely used by physicians who have accepted it as a valuable treatment for vascular disease. This is also its most controversial use. In the past 30 years, I estimate that well over two million patients have been treated with chelation for vascular disease. It has persisted, and the number of doctors administering it has grown dramatically in spite of recurrent attacks by many physicians and organized medical associations over the years. This is unlike many other controversial therapies that have withered in the face of antagonism by opponents of anything outside the mainstream. Membership in the American College for Advancement in Medicine (ACAM), the organization that teaches chelation therapy to physicians, has more than doubled in the past few years to over 1,000 members in 1998. There are practitioners in every state and many foreign countries. Many doctors practice chelation who are not members of ACAM, but the exact number is not known.

CHELATION, FREE RADICALS AND DEGENERATIVE DISEASE

Chelation therapy has many potential health benefits. To understand them you first need to understand something about the underlying pathology of degenerative diseases, including blood vessel diseases affecting the heart, brain and legs, as well as other organs. This pathology is in part the result of excessive "free-radical" activity. Free radicals are unstable, high-energy molecules or fragments of molecules that are missing an electron (electrons in the outer shell of molecules like to be in pairs). In searching for a mate to become stable again, these molecules steal electrons from other molecules, damaging them and generating more free radicals in a chain reaction. The scientific term for this electron theft is oxidation, and free radicals are derived from oxygen. (The opposite reaction, the donation of an electron, is called reduction, and there is an important balance of oxidation and reduction reactions in the body.)

The high energy of free radicals can be put to good use—and many normal metabolic functions depend on them. They can be viewed like sparks in a fireplace, which can warm the house, but if they are in the wrong place—such as the living room rug—they can do a lot of damage, including burning the whole house down. The physiologically important, oxygen-derived free radicals include superoxide and hydroxyl radicals. The hydroxyl radical is the most potent free radical. Singlet oxygen, an excited form of the oxygen we breathe, and peroxides, such as hydrogen peroxide are very high-energy, reactive oxygen species. They readily lead to the formation of free radicals (such as the peroxyl radical), but they are not literally free radicals themselves because they do not have an unpaired electron.[8]

The high energy of ultraviolet light and ionizing radiation can bump an electron out of place, thus creating free radicals. Because of the close relationship between oxidation and free-radical damage, the terms are often used interchangeably, and free-radical protection is referred to as antioxidation. Antioxidant substances help to control the damage from excessive exposure to free radicals. Some free radicals are formed by the combination with nitrogen-based or chlorine-based molecules. They can create a free-radical form of nitric oxide, and a bleach-like compound called hypochlorite.

Although uncontrolled free radicals can be dangerous in excess or in the wrong place, essential free radicals participate in many necessary reactions in the body. Controlled free radicals are important for detoxification, synthesis of major molecules (prostaglandins and melanin), oxidation of metabolites and the transport of electrons. This electron transport is important for energy production in the mitochondria, the little engines that manufacture energy inside cells. Free radicals are also used by the white blood cells as high-energy "bullets" to kill bacteria, viruses and other invading microbes.

It is only when the free radicals get out of hand that they become a problem. They can damage fatty molecules (lipids) in cell membranes and in the bloodstream, and they can disrupt the genetic materials DNA and RNA, in cell nuclei or in the mitochondria, and they can damage other parts of the cell. They can also damage proteins, notably enzymes, by causing denaturation (similar to the congealing of the protein in egg whites when heated) and cross-linking of molecules. All of this damage from free radicals leads to many chronic, degenerative diseases.

Excess exposure to free radicals contributes to the obvious superficial signs of aging, such as wrinkling and loss of elasticity of the skin and the deposition of age pigment (commonly called liver spots). It seems apparent from current research that accelerated internal biological aging is also the result of free-radical damage. Part of the problem is from damage to the mitochondria. Researchers consider free-radical damage to be at the root of many degenerative diseases. Atherosclerosis, cancer, inflammatory joint disease, asthma, diabetes, senile dementia and degenerative eye disease are among them.[9] The cell membrane is important for communication from one cell to another through hormones and regulatory substances called prostaglandins. Disruption of cell membranes interrupts this normal chain of communication and can impair hormonal activity, prostaglandin activity and nerve transmission.

Free radicals are so important in normal metabolism and in destructive processes that it is essential for living organisms to have mechanisms for channeling the necessary free radicals into the right pathways, and for coping with any excess. Our modern environment and lifestyles lead to high levels of exposure to free radicals. Some examples of free radical generators are:

- Environmental pollutants and other industrial chemicals
- Tobacco smoke
- Pesticides
- Oxidized (rancid) or hydrogenated fats
- Medications (indirectly because they activate the liver enzyme called cytochrome p450)
- Inflammation, whether from injury, infection or even allergies
- Transition metals (see below)

Excessive tissue levels of iron appear to be very dangerous. Iron is one of the transition metals that can lead to explosive chain-reaction increases of free-radical production up to a million times what the rate would be without iron present. Iron exists in two energy states (called "ferric" and "ferrous"), and it is the shuttling back and forth between these states that can free up an electron and result in rapid and massive production of free radicals. Note that iron is an essential mineral for health, but high levels may be harmful. Iron tends to accumulate with age, probably due to both dietary and metabolic factors.

Iron excess has been associated with an increased risk of atherosclerosis. Premenopausal women and regular blood donors have some protection from heart disease, and there is evidence that it is the regular loss of iron that provides this protection.[10] Although some investigators have suggested that excess iron storage may simply reflect meat intake, there are other studies that suggest that treatments to reduce iron levels may lower heart disease. Treatment with another chelating agent (desferoxamine), which takes out iron and reduces tissue levels, can decrease free-radical damage to the heart and arteries.[11] In Finland, a large study showed that excess iron storage (as measured by serum ferritin levels) was the most important risk factor for heart disease except for smoking.[12] Meat consumption is very high in Finland and the iron from meat is very well absorbed. Some studies suggest that it is the iron from meat that is more of a problem than total iron intake.[13]

Copper is also a transition metal with two energy states (cupric and cuprous) and in the test tube it can also generate free radicals. However, with copper a deficiency is far more damaging than an excess because copper is an essential cofactor in the activity of superoxide dismutase (SOD), one of the major free-radical scavenger enzymes inside the cells. This enzyme protects cells from free-radical damage. Unlike iron, copper levels tend to decline with age, and one is more likely to see deficiency than excess. Copper excess has not been associated with vascular disease. Chelation patients are routinely given copper supplements as part of the comprehensive protocol.

Antioxidants are produced in the course of normal metabolism to protect tissues, and some are also ingested in the diet. Superoxide dismutase, peroxidases and catalase are produced in the body. Vitamin E, vitamin C, selenium, beta-carotene and flavonoids are antioxidants present in the foods we eat. Coenzyme Q10 is both produced in the body and ingested (but as we age we produce less of it). Sulfur-containing amino acids, such as methionine and glutathione, are also antioxidants. Many of the substances in herbal and botanical medicines act as antioxidants. These antioxidant substances that protect us from free radicals are also called free-radical scavengers. We'll come back to free radicals later, when we discuss the possible mechanisms of action of EDTA chelation therapy, and also during the discussion of antioxidant protection.

EDTA FOR HEAVY METAL TOXICITY

The earliest use for EDTA was in the removal of lead from patients who had accumulated toxic levels. This is common in people who work with lead paint or leaded gasoline, children who live in houses with lead paint and eat the chips from peeling paint, battery workers, industrial workers, artisans who work with leaded glass, and many others. Children do not have to eat the paint chips to become lead toxic; they can simply breathe the dust that is produced by the opening and closing of windows or by the natural erosion of paint over time. Toxic lead exposure is still fairly common today, and the standards for toxicity have been tightened because lead is increasingly being recognized as a toxin at lower levels than previously thought.

Administration of EDTA for heavy metal toxicity is one of the currently accepted uses for this drug. Lead is a neurotoxin and enzyme poison. In addition to the nervous system, lead toxicity harms bone marrow, endocrine glands, kidneys and reproductive systems.[14] These are direct toxic effects rather than free-radical damage. There has been a decline in blood lead levels since the late 1970s, probably as a result of the reduction of the use of lead in gasoline, household paint, food and drink cans, and plumbing systems.[15] However, many people still have significant amounts of lead in their bodies, and the level that is considered toxic continues to be lowered. In 1997, more people than in 1996 had elevated blood lead levels due to occupational lead exposure.[16] This surprised some researchers.

Lead is usually hidden in tissues other than blood; therefore just measuring blood levels is inadequate to determine whether or not your level is high. I had my own lead level checked with a 24-hour urine collection, a standard test, and it showed 17 micrograms (mcg). After an EDTA chelation treatment to pull out hidden lead, the 24-hour level was 113 mcg. This shows that much of the lead is hidden, but can be removed with proper treatment with chelation. (After six treatments my post-treatment 24-hour test showed only 34 mcg, 70 percent less than the first treatment.)

Cadmium is an alkaline earth metal with serious toxicity. It is used industrially, but you may have heard of it mostly through its presence in nickel-cadmium (NiCad) batteries. Cadmium may contribute to high blood pressure[17] and impairment of immune function.[18] One of my patients is an artist who works with pastels, and she inhales the dust from pigments, some of which contain cadmium. She tested very high for cadmium on the 24-hour urine level (20 mcg), but after a series of EDTA treatments her excretion level came down to less than 3 mcg in 24 hours. She had no specific symptoms related to this exposure but she felt that chelation therapy would help prevent problems in the future. EDTA does not remove cadmium very well but it removed enough in this patient to bring her level down below what is considered acceptable.

Other uses of EDTA are in the treatment of severely high blood calcium, abnormal deposits of calcium in inappropriate locations, and heart arrhythmias, including those due to digitalis toxicity. EDTA is not an effective chelating agent for mercury, a highly toxic metal. Although it does bind well with mercury, in the body the mercury appears to be too strongly bound to other molecules such as sulfur groups, or else it is inaccessible to EDTA. Doctors are using other chelating agents for the removal of mercury in patients who are exposed to this metal from industrial sources, paints, fungicides and foods, as well as from dental fillings. DMSA (dimercaptosuccinic acid) is an effective mercury-chelating agent. It is a prescription capsule taken orally, and many doctors recommend it for patients with high mercury or potential risk from numerous amalgam dental fillings.

EDTA FOR VASCULAR DISEASE

By far the most controversial use of EDTA chelation is in the treatment of hardening of the arteries (arteriosclerosis or atherosclerosis), whether cardiac, cerebral or peripheral vascular disease (hardening of the arteries to the heart, brain and legs, respectively). It has been used successfully since the 1950s, but it still remains under a cloud. Although there have been no well-controlled, large-scale, prospective, double-blind studies of chelation therapy, this does not mean that there is no research supporting its use. Numerous smaller studies document the value of chelation in vascular disease.

The truth is that there is a lack of "adequate" scientific research for most medical and surgical treatments that are common today. In fact, there have been no such double-blind studies showing the benefits of bypass surgery. Although it appears to help a few patients, the vast majority of patients who have bypass surgery are operated on unnecessarily. Second opinion studies document this clearly. In one study, 70 percent of patients who asked a cardiologist for a second opinion were told they did not need this very expensive operation.[19] Balloon angioplasty and clot-dissolving drugs have been administered with inadequate documentation for the extent of their use or relative safety. Recent studies are trying to compare the use of medical therapy with balloon angioplasty and bypass surgery, but the answers are not yet clear because therapies are always changing.[20] One research group, noting the widespread use of newly available techniques in cardiology, stated, "Many of these techniques have gained widespread acceptance and use without the benefit of studies demonstrating efficacy."[21]

Many drugs in common use also have inadequate scientific support. Chemotherapy for breast cancer and many other cancers, and many of the drugs used to treat hypertension, are examples of commonly used treatments with inadequate evidence to support their value. Recent reports have suggested that sometimes the drug treatment of moderate levels of hypertension may do more harm than good. Calcium channel blockers can lower blood pressure but the long-term results showed that they did not help mortality. Some of the newer drugs are similarly promoted but we just don't know yet what the results will be. Over-the-counter cold remedies are heavily advertised but there is little evidence that they really help either the patient's symptoms or the cold's duration.

It used to be common practice to administer lidocaine routinely to patients who had just suffered a heart attack. The theory was that irregularities of the heart rhythm commonly caused death, and that lidocaine could reduce arrhythmias. The logic was good but the results—found out sometime later—showed that, except for patients who already had arrhythmias, lidocaine did more harm than good when it was used routinely, rather than only in patients who already had arrhythmias.[22,23] (In other circumstances, lidocaine can be a valuable treatment and it is often added to chelation infusions.)

Estimates by the Congressional Office of Technology Assessment and others suggest that about 85 percent of medical treatments, as they are routinely administered, are not based on adequate scientific studies. This is not necessarily a bad statistic. What it means is that medicine is still an art as well as a science, and as we seek higher levels of scientific support for treatments, we still must treat patients with the best knowledge available. This knowledge includes clinical experience and the experience of colleagues. If we were to wait for absolute scientific support for every medical therapy, physicians would not be able to treat anyone. Currently, the best knowledge we have supports the use of chelation therapy for vascular disease.

In the early 1950s, physicians started to use EDTA chelation for heart disease. Because EDTA binds with calcium, it was their theory that it would remove calcium from plaques in the coronary arteries, and as a result would clear blockages that obstructed the flow of blood in the arteries. This was a logical if simplistic view of the actions of EDTA, but it was in accord with the level of knowledge at the time. What they found was that EDTA chelation did help their patients with angina and other symptoms of vascular disease. Later information has led to a change in the views of how EDTA works for vascular disease, but the research supporting its effectiveness continues to show that it does work.

FOR THE HEART AND OTHER ORGANS

The heart is a muscular pump. Like every other tissue in the body, it requires oxygen to function. The oxygen is carried in the blood by arteries to every tissue. Blood leaves the heart through the largest artery in the body, called the aorta. At the very start of the aorta, where it leaves the heart, small arteries branch off and circle around the heart to supply it with blood. These are the coronary arteries. Other arteries feed all of the body's other tissues and organs. Circulation of life-giving oxygen depends upon these arteries being open. The circulation can be compromised by spasms of muscles in the arterial wall that close the channel, or by an accumulation of substances in the artery that block it. This blockage is called atherosclerosis or arteriosclerosis, or simply hardening of the arteries.

Hardening of the arteries results from repeated damage to the arterial lining cells called endothelium. These cells are akin to the "skin" of the interior artery wall, but they also serve other functions. They produce a substance that helps to relax the muscular wall of the artery and keep the channel open. This substance used to be known by the cumbersome name "endothelial-derived relaxing factor," but is now known as the simple molecule nitric oxide. When an artery goes into spasm as a result of inadequate nitric oxide, it causes reduced blood flow. Damaged endothelial cells can not only lead to decreased blood flow in the short term, but also to local inflammation, infiltration of inflammatory cells, overgrowth of repair tissue and deposits of fat, cholesterol and eventually calcium. This is the developmental process of arteriosclerosis.

A number of lifestyle factors can lead to heart disease. High stress, lack of exercise and high blood pressure contribute to the development of arterial damage. One of the substances that damages arteries is oxidized LDL-cholesterol, the so-called "bad cholesterol." LDL stands for low-density lipoproteins—large fatty-protein molecules that carry cholesterol. They are low-density because their large size prevents them from packing tightly together. This oxidized form of LDL-cholesterol damages the lining cells of the artery walls.

Cholesterol itself is not bad; it is an essential molecule. The "good" HDL-cholesterol (high-density lipoprotein) is an antioxidant free-radical scavenger that can actually protect tissues. The liver produces cholesterol which is the building block for formation of steroid hormones, but when this cholesterol is oxidized it becomes dangerous. The oxidized form is carried more readily in the low-density fraction. Oxidized LDL-cholesterol is one of the culprits in the complex array of events leading to heart and blood vessel disease.[24] Researchers consider that repeated or prolonged attacks on the blood vessel lining by free radicals underlie the development of heart disease. Eventually, the narrowed channels may become acutely blocked with a blood clot, called a thrombosis. In the heart arteries this is called a coronary thrombosis and in the brain a cerebral thrombosis.

The damage that results from blocked arteries depends upon which tissues and organs are being fed by those arteries. Location also determines specific signs and symptoms. For example, blockage in the coronary arteries can lead to fatigue, shortness of breath, and angina pectoris—chest, arm or back pain in response to exertion or stress. It can also lead to a myocardial infarction (heart attack), in which the reduced blood flow is so severe or long lasting that there is death of some heart muscle tissue. Unfortunately for many people, a common initial sign of heart disease is sudden death, which makes prevention much more important than treatment. Later, we'll discuss prevention through lifestyle changes.

FOR THE BRAIN

Blockage in the arteries to the brain can lead to dizziness, impaired memory, loss of vision, balance problems and other altered brain functions. It can occur in the carotid arteries in the neck or in small vessels farther along toward the brain. A transient ischemic attack, or TIA, is a temporary loss of brain function that does not persist long enough to cause permanent damage. This could be from a sudden drop in blood pressure in arteries that are already narrowed. A cerebral infarction (stroke), on the other hand, is the death of brain cells as a result of persistent loss of circulation. It can result from a thrombosis in any of the arteries in the brain, or from a hemorrhage. A hemorrhage most often occurs in vessels that are already fragile as a result of arteriosclerotic damage.

Circulation to the brain also affects vision, as there are many small arteries in the eyes that are affected by arteriosclerosis. Because a physician can see the arteries in the retina through an ophthalmoscope, this examination reveals one of the early signs of hardening of the arteries. Macular degeneration is one of the most devastating conditions occurring in older people. It is loss of the most sensitive area of the retina called the macula, responsible for sharp vision. Chelation therapy has been very effective for many patients to reverse macular degeneration, or at least slow its progression in those who do not respond well.

FOR THE EYES

Paul R., a well-known, modern American figure painter, came to see me in the early 1980s with hypertension. He was on medication but its side effects made him unable to function due to physical fatigue and general lethargy. In addition, the drugs were ineffective at lowering his blood pressure. (He had been told, however, that he could never stop taking his medication.) I put him on a nutrition and dietary supplement program with regular exercise. He stopped taking his medication because he was so exhausted that he was unable to work at painting. In spite of stopping his medication, his blood pressure came down to normal within a matter of weeks.

Paul enjoyed excellent health for a number of years until he noticed an expanding dark spot in the middle of his field of vision in his left eye. As the spot continued to grow, he consulted an eye specialist who diagnosed his condition as a central retinal vein occlusion. He was put in an experimental laser surgery study to see if that could correct the problem. Unfortunately, the surgery was ineffective and he was told that there was no cure for his condition.

Because my previous treatment had proved successful, Paul decided to consult me for this problem in 1991. He was very concerned as he was also told he had a one-in-ten chance of it happening in his other eye, which obviously would have been devastating for a painter. He asked me if chelation might help prevent it from happening. I could not promise that this was the case but he decided to pursue chelation anyway for the possibility of improved circulation to his eyes, and because there was no other treatment being offered. He started on chelation therapy infusions three times a week, and after a few months he recovered about 90 percent of the vision in his left eye. The resultant side benefits were that his additional symptom of painful arthritis in his shoulder joints diminished, and he also experienced improved balance and some restoration of hair color.

Paul stopped chelation after his remarkable recovery and after a few years his vision started to decline again. He started another course of chelation treatments but not as frequently as during his initial therapy. His vision began to recover although only to about 80 percent of the original level. Two years later, his vision started to decline once again after a period of time without chelation, and he has recently restarted therapy with gradual improvement. Paul now realizes that he should try to maintain a regular follow-up program of chelation along with the rest of his health program.

FOR THE ABDOMEN AND LEGS

Peripheral artery disease involves those vessels farther from the heart, mainly to the abdominal organs such as the kidneys, or to the pelvic organs, legs and feet. The kidneys cleanse the blood and their function depends upon good blood flow. Sexual function requires circulation to the pelvic organs, and male sexual dysfunction is a common occurrence when circulation is compromised. If there is poor circulation to the legs, the leg hair stops growing, pulses in the legs and feet are diminished, the skin atrophies and loses color, and open sores appear and won't heal. Eventually, the persistent loss of circulation can lead to gangrene, usually starting with the toes and moving up the leg. This may lead to an amputation of the foot or the leg, depending on the severity of the poor circulation.

PROTOCOL FOR CHELATION THERAPY

The American College for Advancement in Medicine has published a protocol for the safe and effective administration of chelation therapy, first in 1989,[25] and later revised in 1997.[26] The therapy consists of a series of intravenous treatments with EDTA and magnesium, usually mixed in sterile water, dextrose or saline solutions. The number of treatments depends on the severity of the disease and the response of the patient, but usually it is between 20 and 40 treatments over a period of three to four months. Each treatment involves sitting in a recliner chair for up to three or four hours. It is most common for treatments to be given twice a week at the start of therapy but other schedules of treatment, such as one or three times a week, are safe and effective.

In the early days of chelation therapy, starting in the early 1950s, the treatment was administered at a much higher dose than today. It was also administered much more quickly and frequently. When it was realized that this pattern of administration might be harmful to patients with impaired kidney function, both dose and frequency were reduced to safer levels. In spite of very high doses and the inattention to kidney function, there were very few complications. There were, however, some deaths from chelation in those days.

The modern protocol for administration of chelation therapy has thoroughly addressed issues of safety, and there have been no deaths or serious complications from chelation therapy in patients treated with this protocol. Detractors of chelation therapy frequently cite the deaths from chelation over 40 years ago to supposedly demonstrate that chelation can be dangerous. Any treatment that is misused or misunderstood can be dangerous, but when properly administered chelation is one of the safest treatments in medicine. To cite only forty-year-old reports of occasional harm with protocols that are no longer in use shows a clear bias against chelation therapy. Nevertheless, it is important for doctors who want to administer chelation therapy to take a training workshop to learn how to perform it properly, understanding that there is a wide margin of safety for the vast majority of patients.

The protocol recommends at least one day off between treatments to allow the EDTA to clear completely from the bloodstream. (The half-life of EDTA is approximately 45 minutes, meaning that every 45 minutes half of the amount remaining in the body is excreted in the urine.) Because EDTA is virtually completely cleared after one day, however, it is possible to give chelation safely on successive days as long as there is no kidney disease. In this situation it is important for the doctor to monitor kidney function more often, and make sure that there is no change in the blood test for kidney function.

In most cases, the intravenous infusion contains not only EDTA and magnesium, but also other ingredients, some of which are helpful with heart disease and some that make the treatment easier or better tolerated. For example, B vitamins, vitamin C and potassium are often part of the infusion. Sodium bicarbonate is added as a buffer to reduce any irritation of the vein during the infusion, but the irritation is relatively unusual with magnesium in the mixture. Lidocaine, a local anesthetic, is useful for burning or aching at the site of the infusion. It also possesses some potential therapeutic benefits of its own.

A typical dose of EDTA for someone with normal kidney function is three grams (50 mg per kilogram of body weight). Giving this amount over three to four hours (16.67 mg per kg per hour) is a safe rate of administration. Sometimes the treatment is done at half the dose, which can be accomplished in less time. Some chelating doctors feel that the half-dose treatment is as effective as the full dose, but others feel that this lower dose is only one-half to three-fourths as effective.[27] This difference of opinion has not yet been resolved but the historical use has been with the three-gram dose, adjusted for body size and reduced kidney function.

Most physicians with whom I have discussed the issue administer the full dose but they are quite open to the lower dose for patients who are concerned about the amount of time the treatments take. EDTA is water soluble but it does not get inside the cells where there are small organelles, the mitochondria and the nuclei with their membranes. Chelation can protect against free-radical damage to these organelles and lipid membranes if the outside of the cells is bathed for a long enough time which allows the fluids inside and outside the cells to attain equilibrium.

With abnormal kidney function the dose is reduced accordingly to minimize the risk of any side effects. In these patients, the lower dose is administered at a decreased rate of administration over the three-hour period (the dose has been lowered for safety, not time considerations). The concentration of EDTA bathing the cells is more important than the specific dose. With diminished kidney function, the lower dose stays around longer because of lower excretion. The EDTA then bathes the cells at the same level that a higher dose would for a patient with normal kidneys. Careful monitoring of kidney function is a routine part of the chelation protocol. Blood and urine tests are routinely taken before the start of therapy and periodically during the treatment schedule. When given at the proper dose, rate and frequency, EDTA will not harm the kidneys.[28] In many patients, kidney function will improve with chelation because the blood flow through the arteries to the kidneys is enhanced.

Intravenous EDTA treatment is easily performed in a doctor's office without having to go to the hospital. The doctor will require a complete medical evaluation, although if you have had an evaluation from another doctor you may not need everything done again, depending on how thorough the previous exam was, and how recently it was done. In addition, to ensure treatment safety, a variety of blood tests are necessary. Most important is the test for kidney function. If a patient's kidney function is diminished or if there is any question about the safety of the treatment for a particular patient, then testing may be done more frequently. This is up to the doctor to decide. There is almost always a dose of EDTA that the patient will tolerate.

Periodically during the course of EDTA treatments, many doctors will give a vitamin and mineral nutritional intravenous instead of chelation. Chelation removes more than just the toxic metals. It will also remove important nutritional elements such as zinc, manganese, chromium and other trace elements. Although most of the minerals are absorbed when taken orally as supplements, there is an extra measure of safety if the minerals are periodically replaced intravenously. This is often done because the physician is not always sure that the patients are taking the supplements that have been recommended.

If you have chelation therapy, remember to take any supplements that your physician has requested you take. They are very likely important for the safe administration of the chelation, and will prove helpful to you in other ways. The protocol for chelation calls for changes in diet, regular exercise and specific dietary supplements. Later in this guide you will find the specific supplements and dietary guidelines for improving vascular disease and other free-radical diseases.

RESEARCH SUPPORT FOR CHELATION THERAPY

For all of the conditions previously listed as a result of hardening of the arteries, EDTA chelation therapy is a helpful treatment. In addition to vast clinical experience, there is plenty of research to support this conclusion. The results are often dramatic—especially in patients who have been told that they must have surgery or that they carry a "ticking time bomb" in their chest. Often such language is used to intimidate patients into accepting a surgical procedure that they might otherwise reject. If patients did not feel that they were in such a dire emergency situation (and it is rare for heart disease to require emergency surgery), they might feel that they had the time to get a second opinion.

As mentioned previously, second opinions will be against the suggested surgery 70 percent of the time, or more. When asked about chelation instead of other treatments, or as an adjunct to medical therapy, patients are usually told either that: "it won't hurt but it won't help"; "it is unproven"; "it is dangerous"; or even that, "I don't know anything about it except that it does not work." Chelation does have a large body of evidence supporting its value, and recent interest in it is enormous. Increasing numbers of doctors are taking the clinical training and joining the American College for Advancement in Medicine, which teaches doctors about and holds scientific meetings on innovative therapies twice a year.

Research on chelation dates to the early 1950s. The earliest study of EDTA use for treating hardening of the arteries was published in 1956. N.E. Clarke and several colleagues reported on the results of chelation therapy in twenty patients. Nineteen of them improved as measured by physical activity and levels of angina. In six of the patients the electrocardiograms also improved. They stated, "A placebo action seemed improbable for several reasons. There was slight if any clinical improvement until after the discomfort of 20, and with a few, 30 infusions. A patient's progress was based on measured physical activity rather than appraisal of subjective symptoms. The improvement gained has been retained and expanded in all, and in a few for as long as two years. The results have been uniformly good."[29]

Dr. Clarke and his colleagues published another study in 1960 in the *American Journal of Medical Science*.[30] That same year Dr. Clarke published an editorial about their results with chelation in the *American Journal of Cardiology*.[31] In this editorial, he reported that in several hundred patients over a period of several years, "the overall relief from the manifestations of occlusive vascular disease has been superior to that obtained with other methods." They found the best results in patients with diseased arteries in the legs, with "greater ability to walk without the production of pain in the legs . . . increased warmth and improved skin color." In patients with brain disease, they found ". . . relief of vertigo and tinnitus and apparent aid in recovery from acute paralysis, and the signs of senility, even when advanced, have been significantly relieved." In patients with heart disease, he reported ". . . impressive symptomatic relief in 87 percent of a large series of patients with angina pectoris, few recurrences of symptoms and a significant lowering of previously reported mortality rates."

Researchers Meltzer, Ural and Kitchell published a positive report in 1960. Of the ten patients that they studied, nine were significantly better after the treatment.[32] They noted a decrease in the frequency and severity of angina (heart pain on exercise), less need for medication (nitroglycerin for heart pain), greater work capacities and improvement in the electrocardiograms in eight of the patients. It was interesting that the patients demonstrated a cumulative effect from chelation treatments such that, although they did not appear to benefit very much during the course of treatment, after three months they were much improved. The authors concluded that EDTA chelation therapy was very valuable in the treatment of heart disease.

In their follow-up study three years later, the same authors reviewed the patients in the initial study and added 28 new patients to their research.[33] Their conclusion in this paper was that chelation was no better than other therapies for heart disease. This conclusion is inexplicable based upon the data that they presented. E.M. Cranton and J.P. Frackelton analyzed this paper and found that the authors' negative conclusions about chelation were not justified.[34] For example, these were patients with serious heart disease, they received a short course of treatment without follow-up, and after 18 months most of them remained improved, although there were some deaths—not unexpected in such a group. The fact is that, in a group such as this, one would expect progressive deterioration over time, especially since they received no lifestyle or diet counseling, no dietary supplements and no further chelation treatments.

From this report and several more recent reports, it appears that there is consistent misrepresentation of the research in an effort to malign chelation therapy. In between the reports from the fifties to early sixties, and continuing through the nineties, there were numerous small studies reporting the benefits of chelation therapy. The authors found it difficult to have their articles accepted for publication in major journals, but they did publish them in journals that were less well known. This does not mean that the studies are not valuable. They have been consistent in showing benefits from chelation even when they are reported as negative.

In 1964, researcher C.P. Lamar reported on a few patients in whom a variety of vascular diseases improved, including eye disease in diabetics (retinopathy).[35] Although he admitted that the number of patients was small, the results were significant enough to convince him that there was benefit from EDTA chelation. In this article, he cites a 1961 study that appeared in *Lancet* on the safety of chelation in which 2,000 infusions were done without any evidence of kidney toxicity.[36] In 1968, Lamar reported again on nine years of clinical experience with chelation therapy.[37] His results showed improvement in a variety of vascular diseases, including healing of diabetic leg ulcers and retinopathy, macular degeneration and atherosclerotic brain disease.

For some reason, in spite of the numerous studies in the 1950s and 1960s evidencing benefits from chelation, with only one mistakenly reporting that it did not find good results, the reputation of chelation suffered, and little money funded research for this treatment. A number of people think that there must have been some sort of opposition to the treatment that was not based strictly on science. Pharmaceutical and surgical treatments are certainly much more profitable, but there is little apparent evidence of any conspiracy against chelation, although even today it seems that studies with good methodology lose their funding or institutional support for no apparent reason.

The patent on EDTA expired in 1969, further reducing the incentive for pharmaceutical companies to finance the research. Nevertheless, a small group of physicians maintained an interest in chelation therapy and continued to treat patients, teach other doctors and do research. One such research paper was published in the *Journal of Holistic Medicine* in 1981 on treating heart disease with chelation therapy.[38] The researcher, Dr. Casdorph, measured the strength of the heart muscle before and after 20 treatments with EDTA in 18 patients who had documented heart disease. The strength of the heart muscle is a reflection of the overall health of the heart and its ability to pump out the blood that comes into it. The average improvement in this "ejection fraction" was just under six percent, which was highly statistically significant.

That same year, the same author in the same journal published another study on 15 patients with impaired cerebral blood flow.[39] He used a technetium-99 brain-flow study, which showed statistically significant improvements in cerebral blood flow in almost all of the patients. What may have been more important for the patients was their clinical improvement in symptoms such as confusion, delusional thinking, dizziness, vertigo, post-stroke paralysis and memory loss (even in those without objective evidence of blood-flow improvement). The patients received between 13 and 26 treatments, most of them having 20 infusions.

In 1982, McDonagh, Rudolph and Cheraskin studied 57 patients with reduced cerebral blood flow as measured by ocular pulse pressure, a noninvasive technique to evaluate the pressure in the eye's ophthalmic artery.[40] The method compares this pressure with the blood pressure in the arm and gives a good reflection of the amount of blockage of blood flow in the carotid arteries. These patients received between 10 and 46 treatments with EDTA chelation. The measurement after therapy showed an average decline in blockage of 18 percent, which was highly significant—less than one in a thousand probability that the result was due to chance. Eighty-eight percent of these patients improved with the therapy.

In 1983, Casdorph and Farr reported on improvement in blood flow in the legs with chelation therapy.[41] In four patients, arteriosclerosis had progressed to such an extent that they experienced atrophy of the skin of the lower legs plus nonhealing and gangrenous ulcerations on the toes and feet such that amputation had already been recommended. All four patients were spared amputation, and one year after treatment they remained healed with intact extremities and no pain. In one of the cases, a measure of the pulse volume in the toe called a plethysmograph showed the return of a pulse where none was detected at the start of therapy.

Throughout the 1980s, McDonagh and Rudolph published a number of papers on the effects of chelation therapy on various health parameters, including cholesterol levels, kidney function, heart, brain and leg circulation, fatigue, and general medical problems as reflected in an extensive questionnaire. The results have been uniformly favorable. More recently, studies have been done in other centers confirming the value of chelation therapy, and criticism of chelation has been inaccurate and biased.

In Brazil, Drs. Olszewer and Carter studied nearly 3,000 subjects with a variety of chronic degenerative diseases, mainly vascular disease. They published their results in 1988, showing that almost 90 percent of patients improved with chelation therapy as measured by changes in their cardiograms, their ability to walk, and Doppler testing of their legs.[42] They followed this with a small, double-blind study that showed improvement in blockages to the legs as measured—again—by walking distance and also by measurement of pressure in the vessels to the legs.[43]

Dr. Guillermo Escobar and his colleagues in Mexico studied vascular disease of the legs in 80 patients and published their results in a surgery journal.[44] Ninety-four percent of patients improved using the therapy by objective testing. Once again, the results were highly significant with less than one in a thousand probability that they could be due to chance alone.

A meta-analysis is a review of studies. It involves taking a collection of studies and seeing if their combined results provide a further clue to the effectiveness of a treatment when any one of the studies alone might be inadequate to prove the therapy's value. Drs. Terry Chappell and John Stahl published a meta-analysis of chelation therapy in 1993.[45] In the 19 studies that they included in their analysis, they gathered data on a total of 22,765 patients. Their statistics showed an 88 percent likelihood that the treatment was effective, with 87 percent of the patients improving overall.

This is a comprehensive view of chelation therapy and presents an emphatic summary of the benefits of the treatment.

Two Danish doctors, Claus Hancke and Knut Flytlie, published a study of 470 patients in 1993.[46] They showed an improvement in between 80 and 91 percent of patients, depending upon which measurement they used. Most importantly, of the 92 patients who had been told they had to have surgery, only 10 ended up requiring the operation. Twenty-four out of twenty-seven legs were saved from amputation. During the entire study they saw no serious side effects or casualties from the treatment.

More recently, a respected surgeon, Dr. John Olwin, affiliated with the Department of Surgery, Rush Presbyterian-St. Luke's Medical Center, in Chicago, Illinois, reported on the use of chelation therapy to treat vascular disease. His article discusses the rationale for the treatment, including the benefits from two of the other ingredients in the infusion—magnesium and heparin.[47] Again, his conclusion is that the weight of evidence favors the use of chelation therapy not only for the treatment of cardiovascular disease, but also for prevention. The authors conclude ". . . there is an impressive body of scientific evidence to support its use both as a prophylactic and active therapy. Further large-scale controlled clinical trials will be critical in convincing the medical community about the cardiovascular benefits of chelation therapy."

In spite of all the favorable articles on chelation therapy, however, there have been two studies in the past few years that purported to show that chelation therapy was ineffective. A close examination of these studies reveals flaws in the design, execution and reporting of the results. Vascular surgeons were the investigators in both of the studies. A Danish study published in two journals did not follow the current protocol for chelation therapy, even though the authors claimed that they did.[48,49] They treated mainly smokers who, generally, do not respond as well to treatment because of their ongoing exposure to free radicals. This study was severely criticized by the Danish Committee on Scientific

Dishonesty.[50] In spite of the faults with the study, the treatment did appear to have some benefits.

The second study took place in New Zealand, and it indicated benefits from chelation therapy with significant improvement in walking distance in patients with hardening of the arteries to the legs.[51] The so-called placebo group was also given active ingredients, as opposed to a real placebo, which is supposed to be totally inactive. Nevertheless, the group receiving the EDTA did far better than the control group when the statistics were evaluated properly. This was in spite of the fact that the subjects were mostly smokers. A letter to the editor in the *New Zealand Medical Journal* reported the correct analysis of this data.[52] Unfortunately, the authors of this study drew incorrect conclusions from the data, which damaged the reputation of chelation in the minds of many doctors who read the conclusions but not the study. Detractors of chelation have used both this and the Danish study to "prove" that it is of no value. When the entire weight of the evidence is reviewed chelation is clearly proven to be beneficial.

The overall picture of chelation therapy is that of a safe, effective therapy for a variety of conditions related to circulation problems and metal toxicity. But these are not the only benefits from chelation therapy. Chelation apparently reduces the risk of developing many chronic diseases, especially those related to free-radical damage or metal toxicity. Among other possible conditions, free radicals have been implicated in causing cancer, inflammatory joint disease, asthma, diabetes, senile dementia and degenerative eye disease.[53] Patients who were treated with chelation in Switzerland between 1958 and 1976 had a far lower incidence of cancer than did other subjects in the same community in Switzerland who did not receive the treatment.[54]

The *Journal of Cardiovascular Nursing* asked me to write an article which would review the literature on chelation in order for them to present a view to their readers that was more comprehensive than the glib rejection of chelation that they would commonly read in editorials. Dr. Terry Chappell and I reviewed the historical use and scientific support for chelation therapy, showing its many benefits and great potential as a medical therapy, and we were being somewhat conservative at the journal editor's request.[55] The only criticism of this article that I have seen was on the Internet, and the comment was that it was "published in an obscure nursing journal."

In 1996, a very favorable review of chelation with magnesium-EDTA was finally published in *Cardiovascular Drug Therapy,* a standard medical textbook.[56] In his introductory comments, Martin Rubin, Ph.D., a researcher with a long history of understanding the importance of chelation in the management of heart disease, states the situation elegantly: "The complex pathophysiologic cascade of the development of atherosclerosis, with its major stages of lipid oxidation initiating vascular wall damage, ensuing coagulation, and underlying cell death with calcification, poses a therapeutic challenge. That these individual processes exist simultaneously at varied sites limits the applicability of therapeutic agents targeted to one or another component of the disease progression. In this respect, EDTA chelation therapy has an implicit advantage in that it can favorably influence all facets of the disease development." He goes on to describe the chemistry, metabolism and therapeutic applications of EDTA chelation therapy. That this appeared in a cardiovascular textbook on drug therapy was revolutionary.

The emergence of coronary bypass surgery with the increasing sophistication of the heart-lung pump certainly made this approach to heart disease more glamorous than simple, safe, inexpensive intravenous therapy. Thinking that the plumbing could be fixed by taking a mechanical approach to the human body seemed straightforward, but we now know that the body is not so simple, and heart disease is not so easily managed with surgery. Although not as high-tech, noninvasive treatments and lifestyle approaches to health appear to be superior to medical or surgical treatment for many patients.[57]

SAFETY AND COSTS OF CHELATION THERAPY

The safety of chelation is far superior to coronary artery bypass surgery. Since the 1950s, with millions of treatments given, there have been no serious side effects when the treating physician has followed the currently accepted protocol. When the Food and Drug Administration collaborated in efforts to perform new studies on chelation in the late 1980s, they bypassed any further safety studies on EDTA because they recognized its low risk. (These research efforts have been blocked at various steps so far, but they and other research projects are ongoing in the late 1990s. Why these studies have not been completed is a subject for a political book rather than a health book.)

On the other hand, the mortality from coronary bypass operations can be quite high depending on the age of the patient and which surgical team is performing the surgery.[58,59] Bypassed arteries do close up again, sometimes within months and commonly within seven years after surgery—and the bypassed arteries close up faster than they would have otherwise.[60] Although some centers have a better surgical record than others, the chances are that you will not have the best; that goes against the law of averages which suggests you are most likely to get an average surgeon.

A coronary artery bypass operation can cost upwards of $50,000, depending upon how many vessels are bypassed while a course of 30 chelation treatments might run about $3,000. The fees for chelation vary in the U.S. from about $65 in some communities to $120 in others. With medical visits and testing the total cost can reach $4–5,000. Unfortunately, most insurance companies do not cover chelation therapy. I have had many patients who were scheduled for bypass surgery, which would have been completely covered by the insurance company, but they were unable to get reimbursement for the safer treatment that cost about one-tenth as much and worked for these patients.

HOW DOES CHELATION WORK?

We don't know for sure how chelation works, however, there are many plausible theories. The fact is that the exact mechanisms by which chelation produces its beneficial effects in degenerative diseases is not certain, but there are many actions of EDTA which might account for some of the improvements. Free-radical reduction/antioxidation is currently the leading candidate for the most important effect of EDTA chelation due to its removing metallic catalysts.[61] Removal of heavy metals can also account for some of the benefits of chelation because of their direct toxicity to many enzyme systems.

EDTA also binds with calcium in the bloodstream, and will reduce the influx of calcium into cells in favor of magnesium. The accumulation of calcium within cells, a common occurrence with aging, damages enzyme systems. EDTA helps magnesium get into the cells partly by blocking calcium. Magnesium acts as a relaxant for blood vessels and this in itself can help to improve blood flow. EDTA also affects hormones and prostaglandins and it has a direct effect in preventing the oxidation of LDL-cholesterol. Chelation also has some antiplatelet and anticoagulant effects, both of which can help vascular disease.

With many possible beneficial actions resulting from EDTA chelation, and the numerous clinical studies that indicate it does work, it is important that research continue on clinical effects and specific actions. In the meantime, for patients with heart disease it is logical for them to look into chelation therapy in an effort to reduce their use of medication—and definitely before they agree to surgery. It is also wise to consider chelation for preventive medicine, especially if you have a family history of heart disease or have not followed a healthy lifestyle.

GUIDELINES FOR THE CHELATION PATIENT

SUPPLEMENTS TO TAKE

Dietary supplements play two roles for patients having chelation therapy. First, they are important to ensure the safety of chelation which otherwise might deplete the body of certain nutrients. Second, many of them are therapeutic themselves, and they can help prevent recurrence of the vascular disease being treated. Most important are the mineral supplements. Many minerals are removed by chelation and they must be replaced. Zinc depletion may lead to a skin rash; zinc is also a cofactor in the activity of the enzyme SOD in the mitochondria. (SOD is important for free-radical control.) It is typical for chelation patients to take 30 mg of zinc daily, and many times an extra 30–50 mg is recommended. Sometimes patients with very low zinc may be asked to take more but zinc competes with copper, and too much zinc can reduce copper levels. Low copper can impair the activities of SOD in the cytoplasm.

Manganese is another mineral that we need to replace for chelation patients because it is readily removed by the treatment. In fact, it is probably more effectively removed than any other nutrient mineral. I usually recommend 20 mg of manganese daily. Manganese is another cofactor for the activity of SOD—the SOD that is active in the mitochondria.

Chelation therapy can deplete the body's supply of vitamin B6, or pyridoxine, and a deficiency can again lead to a skin rash. When skin rashes do occur it is usually because patients are not taking their recommended amounts of pyridoxine and zinc. It is common to give about 100 mg of pyridoxine to patients—but with caution. Very high doses of pyridoxine have been rarely associated with a peripheral neuropathy (numbness and tingling of the arms and hands with some loss of function). When given in balance with other nutrients, including magnesium, it is unusual for pyridoxine to cause problems. I have given pyridoxine for over 20 years, and only in one patient did I ever see a problem. For reasons she could never explain, she was taking about 3,000 mg daily, thinking that it would help her neuropathy which only continued to get worse. Pyridoxine has recently been shown to help reduce homocysteine levels (a metabolite associated with heart disease).[62] Independent of its association with homocysteine, for reasons not yet explained, a low pyridoxine level has been associated with an increased incidence of atherosclerosis.[63]

Magnesium is so important to the heart that every chelation patient takes it as a supplement even though it is part of the intravenous infusion. The typical dose of magnesium is between 500 and 1,000 mg per day. Many other nutrients help vascular disease and are commonly part of the therapy for chelation patients. The supplements and their daily doses include coenzyme Q10 (100–400 mg), vitamin C (4,000–8,000 mg), vitamin E (800–1,200 IU), L-carnitine (500–2,000 mg), L-lysine (1,000–1,500 mg), and deodorized garlic (500–5,000 mg). A nutritionally oriented physician may recommend many other nutrients, flavonoids or botanicals that are too extensive to go into in more detail here. Many of them are excellent antioxidants and have their own therapeutic value.

DIET AND LIFESTYLE CHANGES THAT HELP

Having chelation therapy for vascular disease and taking supplements does not mean that someone can continue in the unhealthy lifestyle that most likely led to the problem in the first place. Because diet is something that can be controlled, changing it allows participation in a very powerful therapeutic activity. I recommend a mostly vegetarian, whole-foods diet. As much as possible, avoid added sugar, white flour, margarine and other hydrogenated oils, and commercially processed oils, as well as artificial flavors, colors and preservatives. I also caution patients to be careful about caffeine consumption in coffee and tea. Caffeine is a stimulant and has been associated with an increased risk of heart disease among other problems.

Most of the existing scientific literature indicates that a plant-based diet is healthier than one with a lot of animal products. The staples of a healthy diet are high fiber foods such as whole grains, fresh vegetables, fruits and legumes. Cultures where these are the habitual foods exhibit very little heart disease and a very low incidence of other diseases related to a rich, refined-food, western diet. Colon cancer and other cancers, varicose veins, hemorrhoids, diabetes and hypertension are the product of lifestyle, not genetics. Diet and exercise are part of this lifestyle. If you are getting chelation therapy, consider helping your own care by following the best health program you can.

It is important to maintain a regular program of physical activity not only for cardiovascular health, but also for many other immediate and long-term health benefits. For example, there is evidence that physical fitness reduces mortality from all causes.[64] In this study, men and women at the lowest level of fitness based upon treadmill tests had a much higher mortality rate than those at the highest levels of fitness, when the results were adjusted for age. Another study showed that people of both sexes and at all ages had a lower mortality from all causes—and specifically from heart disease—if they had a lower resting heart rate.[65] Physical fitness tends to lower the resting heart rate. Exercise also reduces cancer mortality and the frequency of adult-onset diabetes.

Stress management has also been associated with lower rates of heart disease, lower blood pressure and many other health benefits. You can easily incorporate relaxation techniques such as meditation, yoga, breathing exercises, visualization and prayer into your lifestyle. They take some time but they do not have to dominate your schedule to be effective. Even a few moments of closing your eyes and imagining you are away on vacation in a tropical island can be very relaxing. Incorporating many of these lifestyle enhancements will help to ensure that you get the best results from your chelation treatment. No treatment for a condition with the progressive nature of heart and vascular diseases is permanent, so you need to make lifestyle changes for your long-term health.

CONCLUSION

EDTA chelation therapy clearly helps in the treatment of metal toxicity, and in general in the reduction of free-radical damage and related diseases. As such, it may very well be one of the best preventive medicine therapies available along with antioxidant dietary supplements; chelation with EDTA is also one of the most valuable, safest and least expensive treatments for heart and blood vessel disease. Heart and blood vessel diseases are the number one killers in the United States and many other industrialized nations. We must look at every avenue for the best treatments.

The usual treatments, such as coronary bypass surgery and balloon angioplasty, are expensive and carry significant risk. They have not yet been shown to be of clear benefit for the majority of patients. If you need treatment for vascular disease it is important to consider the value of chelation therapy, which has so many direct and side benefits with so few negative side effects. It would be well worth your while to find a doctor who performs chelation therapy as part of a comprehensive approach to treatment. You can find a physician in your area by calling the American College for Advancement in Medicine at 800–532–3688 or visiting their website at www.acam.org. Incorporate all of the lifestyle changes that have proven so valuable as additional measures by which you can help yourself. The most important approach you can take is to make an informed decision.

REFERENCES

1. Perry Jr. HM, Schroeder HA, "Depression of cholesterol levels in human plasma following ethyleene diamine tetra acetate and hydralazine." *J Chronic Dis* 1955 Nov; 2(5):520–533.
2. Peters HA, "Trace minerals, chelating agents and the porphyrias." *Fed Proc* 1961 Sept; 20 #3 (Part II Supp. #10):227–234.
3. Woods SM, Peters JA, Johnson SAM "Chelation therapy in cutaneous porphyria." *Arch Derm* 1961 Dec; 84:82–89.
4. Neldner KE, Winkelmann, RK, Perry, H, "Scleroderma." *Arch Derm* 1962 Sept; 86:95–99.
5. Birk RE, "Treatment of systemic sclerosis." *Modern Treatment* 1966 Nov; 3(6):1287–1301.
6. Cranton, EM, 1988, personal communication with author.
7. Leipzig LJ, Boyle AJ, McCann DS, "Case histories of rheumatoid arthritis treated with sodium or magnesium EDTA." *J Chron Dis* 1970; 22:553–563.
8. Halstead BW, Rozema TC, *The Scientific Basis of EDTA Chelation Therapy,* Landrum, South Carolina: TRC Publishing, 1997.
9. Florence TM, "The role of free radicals in disease." *Aust N Z J Ophthalmol* 1995 Feb; 23(1):3–7.
10. Meyers DG, Strickland D, Maloley PA, Seburg JK, Wilson JE, McManus BF, "Possible association of a reduction in cardiovascular events with blood donation." *Heart* 1997 Aug; 78(2):188–193.
11. Katoh S, Toyama J, Kodama I, Akita T, Abe T, "Desferoxamine, an iron chelator, reduces myocardial injury and free-radical generation in isolated neonatal rabbit hearts subjected to a global ischaemia-reperfusion." *J Molec Cell Cardiology* 1992; 24:1267–1275.

12. Salonen JT, Nyyssonen K, Korpela H, Tuomilehto J, Seppanen R, Salonen R, "High stored iron levels are associated with excess risk of myocardial infarction in eastern Finnish men." *Circulation* 1992 Sept; 86(3):803–811.
13. Asherio A, Willett WC, Rimm EB, Giovannucci EL, Stampfer MJ, "Dietary iron intake and risk of coronary disease among men." *Circulation* 1994 Mar; 89(3):969–974.
14. Agency for Toxic Substances and Disease Registry, "Toxicological profile for lead." Atlanta, Georgia: U.S. Department of Health and Human Services, Public Health Service, 1993; publication no. PB93–182475.
15. Centers for Disease Control, Preventing Lead Poisoning in Young Children: A Statement by the Centers for Disease Control. Altanta, Georgia: U.S. Department of Health and Human Services, Public Health Service, 1991.
16. Ibid. *Morbidity and Mortality Weekly Reports,* 1998; 47:77–80.
17. Schroeder HA, "Possible relationships between trace metals and chronic diseases." *Metal-Binding in Medicine,* 132, Seven MJ (Ed), 1960. Philadelphia: J.B. Lippincott, 59–67.
18. Halstead BW, Rozema TC, *The Scientific Basis of EDTA Chelation Therapy,* Landrum, South Carolina: TRC Publishing, 1997.
19. Graboys TB, Biegelsen B, Lampert S, Blatt CM, Lown B, "Results of a second-opinion program for coronary artery bypass grafting surgery." *JAMA* 1987; 259:1611–1614.
20. Solomon AJ, Gersh BJ, "Management of chronic stable angina: medical therapy, percutaneous transluminal coronary angioplasty, and coronary artery bypass graft surgery. Lessons from the randomized trials." *Ann Int Med* 1998 Feb. 1; 128(3):216–223.
21. Goldberg RJ, Gore JM, Dalen JE, "Current practice patterns in the management of acute myocardial infarction." Survey of the American College of Chest Physicians. *Chest* 1987 Sept; 92(3):550–554.
22. Tisdale JE, "Lidocaine prophylaxis in acute myocardial infarction." *Henry Ford Hospital Medical Journal* 1991; 39(3–4):217–225.
23. Hargarten K, et al. "Prehospital prophylactic lidocaine does not favorably affect outcome in patients with chest pain." *Ann Emerg Med* 1990 Nov; 19(11):1274–1279.
24. Steinberg D, "Antioxidants and atherosclerosis, a current assessment." *Circulation* 1991 Sept; 84(3):1420–1425.
25. Cranton EM, "Protocol of the American College of Advancement in Medicine for the safe and effective administration of

EDTA chelation therapy." *J Adv Med* 1989 Spring/Summer; 2(1/2):269–305.

26. Rozema TC, "Protocol for the safe and effective administration of EDTA and other chelating agents for vascular disease, degenerative disease, and metal toxicity." *J Adv Med* 1997 Spring; 10(1):5–100.
27. Cranton EM, 1997 Dec, personal communication with author.
28. McDonagh EW, Rudolph CJ, Cheraskin E, "The effect of EDTA chelation therapy plus supportive multivitamin-trace mineral supplementation upon renal function: a study in serum creatinine. *J Holist Med* 1982; 4:146.
29. Clarke NE, Clarke CN, Mosher RE, "Treatment of angina pectoris with disodium ethylene diamine tetraacetic acid." *Am J of Med Sci* 1956 Dec:654–666.
30. ibid. 1960. "Treatment of occlusive vascular disease with ethylenediaminetetraacetic acid." *Am J of Med Sci* 1960;239:732.
31. Clarke NE, "Atherosclerosis, occlusive vascular disease and EDTA." *Am J Cardiol* 1960 Aug; 1(2):233–236.
32. Meltzer LE, Ural E, Kitchell JR, "The treatment of coronary artery heart disease with disodium EDTA." *Metal-Binding in Medicine*, 132, Seven MJ (Ed), 1960 Philadelphia: J.B. Lippincott.
33. Kitchell JR, Palmon F, Aytan N, Meltzer LE, "The treatment of coronary artery disease with disodium EDTA, a reappraisal." *Am J Cardiol* 1963; 11:501–506.
34. Cranton EM, Frackelton JP, "Current status of EDTA chelation therapy in occlusive arterial disease." *J Adv Med* 1989 Spring/Summer; 2(1/2):107–119.
35. Lamar CP, "Chelation therapy of occlusive arteriosclerosis in diabetic patients." *Angiology* 1964; 15:379–394.
36. Meltzer LE, Palmon FP, Kitchell JR, "Hypoglycemia induced by disodium ethylenediamine tetraacetic acid," *Lancet* 1961; 2(7203):637.
37. Lamar CP, "Calcium chelation in atherosclerosis: nine years clinical experience new modus operandi." American College of Angiology, 14th Annual Meeting, 1968 Dec 3–8.
38. Casdorph HR, "EDTA chelation therapy: efficacy in arteriosclerotic heart disease." *J Holist Med* 1981; 3:53–59.
39. *ibid.* "EDTA chelation therapy II: efficacy in brain disorders." *J Holist Med* 1981; 3:101–117.
40. McDonagh EW, Rudolph CJ, Cheraskin E, "An oculocerebrovasculometric analysis of the improvement in arterial stenosis following EDTA chelation therapy." *J Holist Med* 1982 Spring/Summer; 4(1):21–23.

41. Casdorph HR, Farr CH, "EDTA chelation therapy: treatment of peripheral arterial occlusion, an alternative to amputation." *J Holist Med* 1983 Spring/Summer; 5(1):3–15.
42. Olszewer E, Carter JP, "EDTA chelation therapy in chronic degenerative disease." *Med Hypoth* 1988; 27:41–49.
43. Olszewer E, Sabbag FC, Carter JP, "A pilot double-blind study of sodium-magnesium EDTA in peripheral vascular disease." *J Nat Med As* 1990; 82:173–177.
44. Escobar GA, Escobar, SC, Ordonez I, Gonzalez M, "Cirugia y Cirujanos" (Surgery and Surgeons), 1995; 61,No.2:58–62 (Mexico).
45. Chappell LT, Stahl JP, "The correlation between EDTA chelation therapy and improvement in cardiovascular function: a meta-analysis." *J Adv Med* 1993; 6:139–160.
46. Hancke C, Flytlie K, "Benefits of EDTA chelation therapy in arteriosclerosis: a retrospective study of 470 patients." *J Adv Med* 1993 Fall; 6(3):161–171.
47. Olwin JH, et al. "Rationale for the use of EDTA-magnesium-heparin therapy in subjects with coronary artery disease." *J Adv Med* 1997 Summer; 10(2):105–128.
48. Sloth-Nielsen J, Guldager B, Mouritzen C, et al. "Arteriographic findings in EDTA chelation therapy on peripheral arteriosclerosis." *Am J Surg* 1991; 162:122–125.
49. Guldager B, Jelnes R, Jorgensen SJ, et al. "EDTA treatment of intermittent claudication—a double-blind, placebo-controlled study." *J Int Med* 1992; 231:261–267.
50. The Committee on Scientific Dishonesty (UVVU), Danish Research Councils, Conclusion concerning complaints in connection with trial of EDTA versus placebo in the treatment of arteriosclerosis. 40 HC Andersens Boulevard, 1553 Kobbenhaven, Denmark.
51. Van Rij AM, Solomon C, Packer SGK, Hopkins WG, "Chelation therapy for intermittent claudication: a double-blind, randomized, controlled trial." *Circulation* 1994; 90:1194–1199.
52. Godfrey ME, Chappell LT, Letter to the editor. *NZMJ* 1996 Mar 6; 109:83.
53. Florence TM, "The role of free radicals in disease." *Aust N Z J Ophthalmol.* 1995 Feb; 23(1):3–7.
54. Blumer W, Cranton EM, "Ninety percent reduction in cancer mortality after chelation therapy with EDTA." *J Adv Med* 1989 Spring/Summer; 2(1/2):183–188.
55. Chappell LT, Janson M, "EDTA chelation therapy in the treatment of vascular disease." *J Cardiovasc Nurs.* 1996 Apr; 10(3):78–86.

56. *Cardiovascular Drug Therapy,* 2nd ed., Messerli FH (ed.) Philadelphia: W.B. Saunders, 1996.
57. Ornish D, Brown SE, "Can lifestyle changes reverse coronary heart disease?" *Lancet* 1990; 366:129.
58. CASS Principal Investigators and the Associates: Coronary Artery Surgery Study (CASS): A randomized trial of coronary artery bypass surgery: Survival data. *Circulation* 1983; 68:939–950.
59. Edmunds LH, Stephenson LW, Edie RN, Ratcliffe MB, "Open-heart surgery in octogenarians." *N Eng J Med.* 1988; 319:131–136.
60. Cashin WL, Sanmarco ME, Nessim SA, Blankenhorn DH, "Accelerated progression of atherosclerosis in coronary vessels with minimal lesions that are bypassed." *N Eng J Med* 1984; 311:824–828.
61. Cranton EM, Frackelton JP, "Free radical pathology in age-associated diseases: treatment with EDTA chelation, nutrition and antioxidants." *J Adv Med* 1989 Spring/Summer; 2(1/2):17–54.
62. Selhub, J, et al. "Association between plasma homocysteine concentrations and extracranial carotid-artery stenosis." *N Eng J Med.* 1995 Feb 2; 332(5):286–291.
63. Robinson K, et al. "Low vitamin B6 or folate levels associated with atherosclerosis." *Circulation* 1998; 97:437–443.
64. Blair SN, Kohl HW, Paffenbarger RS Jr., Clark DG, Cooper KH, Gibbons LW, "Physical fitness and all-cause mortality. A prospective study of healthy men and women." *JAMA* 1989 Nov. 3; 262(17):2395–2401.
65. Kannel WB, Kannel C, Paffenbarger RS Jr., Cupples, LA, "Heart rate and cardiovascular mortality: the Framingham Study." *Am Heart J.* 1987 June; 113(6):1489–1494.